OPTIMAL KETO DIET FOOD LIST

Fuel Your Ketogenic Journey With The Ultimate Food Arsenal

Garrick Goldner

All Rights Reserved

Without express explicit consent from the author or the publisher, the information in this book may not be copied, duplicated, or transferred. Under no circumstances will the publisher or author be held accountable or held legally liable for any losses, expenses, or damages resulting directly or indirectly from the information included in this book.

Legal Notice

This book is covered by copyright. It is solely meant for private use. Without the author's or publisher's permission, no portion of this work may be changed, distributed, sold, used, quoted, or paraphrased.

Disclaimer Notice

Please be aware that the material in this booklet is only intended for informational and recreational use. Every attempt has been made to provide accurate, current, trustworthy, and comprehensive information. However, there are no express nor implied guarantees of any sort. Readers recognize that the author is not offering expert advice in law, finance, medicine, or other related fields. This book's information came from a variety of sources. Before using any strategies described in this book, please seek the advice of a qualified specialist. By reading this book, the reader acknowledges that the author shall not be liable for any direct or indirect damages arising from using the information herein, including, but not limited to, mistakes, omissions, or inaccuracies.

TABLE OF CONTENTS

TABLE OF CONTENTS ii

WHAT ARE THE FOOD OPTIONS AVAILABLE ON A KETOGENIC DIET? 1

IS THE KETOGENIC DIET BENEFICIAL FOR YOUR HEALTH? 4

WHAT ARE THE EFFECTS OF KETO FLU ON YOUR BODY? 7

VEGETABLES 11

LEAFY GREENS 15

FATS 18

FRUITS 20

MEATS AND POULTRY 23

SEAFOOD 25

NUTS AND SEEDS 27

PLANT-BASED PROTEINS 29

DAIRY AND EGGS 31

BEVERAGES 33

FLOURS FOR BAKING 36

SWEETENERS 38

HERBS AND SPICES 40

CONDIMENTS 42

CONCLUSION 44

Introduction To Optimal Keto Diet Food List

A ketogenic diet involves primarily consuming fats, a moderate amount of protein, and minimal carbohydrates. In a strict ketogenic diet, carbohydrates contribute only 5% of the overall energy, despite the body's natural preference for them.

By reducing carbohydrate intake, the body enters a state called ketosis. In this state, the body breaks down fat and utilizes ketone bodies for energy since it lacks the usual supply of blood sugar from carbohydrates. However, certain cells in your body will still absorb carbohydrates and use them as an energy source once you enter ketosis.

In the past, ketogenic diets were mainly prescribed to patients with epilepsy. However, extensive research has been conducted to explore the potential benefits of this diet in the treatment of cancer, diabetes, polycystic ovary syndrome (PCOS), obesity, excessive cholesterol, and cardiovascular disease. Additionally, many individuals choose ketogenic diets as a means of weight loss.

If you're considering transitioning from a high-carbohydrate, moderate-protein, high-fat diet to a low-carbohydrate, low-fat diet and are unsure where to begin, it's understandable to feel overwhelmed. Adopting a ketogenic diet involves planning your meals, avoiding certain foods, and occasionally indulging in specific food items.

To grasp all the details, it is important to read and understand the information thoroughly.

WHAT ARE THE FOOD OPTIONS AVAILABLE ON A KETOGENIC DIET?

Certainly! The keto diet offers a wide range of real and nourishing food options that align with its low-carb principles. This way of eating emphasizes the consumption of seafood, meat, vegetables, healthy fats, and fresh fruits. These ingredients provide essential nutrients and help keep you satiated while providing sustained energy throughout the day.

One of the benefits of the keto diet is that you can still enjoy indulgent and comforting foods, albeit with a few modifications. Thanks to the availability of keto-friendly flours and powders, preparing snacks that align with the dietary guidelines has become more convenient. You can find alternatives for traditional high-carb ingredients, allowing you to create delicious low-carb versions of your favorite treats.

It's important to note that while occasional indulgence is possible on the keto diet, it's crucial to avoid sweets and high-carb snacks on a regular basis. These items typically contain unhealthy fats, high sugar content, and refined carbohydrates, which can contribute to weight gain, elevated blood sugar levels, and increased cholesterol. By sticking to the principles of the keto diet and focusing on whole, unprocessed foods, you can optimize your health and achieve your weight loss goals.

It's essential to approach the keto diet with patience and dedication. Weight loss progress may vary from person to person, but by consistently adhering to the diet and making healthy choices, you can experience positive results over time. It's worth noting that the keto diet is not just about weight loss but also offers potential benefits for overall health and well-being, such as improved insulin sensitivity and increased mental clarity.

By focusing on real, low-carb foods and making mindful choices, you can enjoy a wide variety of delicious meals and snacks while reaping the potential benefits of the keto lifestyle.

IS THE KETOGENIC DIET BENEFICIAL FOR YOUR HEALTH?

A ketogenic diet, when followed diligently, can be considered safe for many individuals. However, it is crucial to consult with a healthcare professional, such as a doctor, qualified nutritionist, or dietitian, before embarking on such a regimen. Their expertise can help identify any potential nutritional deficiencies or other health implications that may arise.

Research findings suggest that low-carb diets, including the ketogenic diet, can offer benefits for individuals with certain medical conditions and aid in appetite control. For example, ketogenic diets have been recommended as a treatment for epileptic seizures in some cases, particularly in children who are unresponsive to medication.

However, there is an ongoing debate among researchers about the long-term effects of low-carb diets on overall nutrition, especially for individuals with pre-existing liver, pancreatic, or gallbladder issues. In these cases, it becomes even more important to seek guidance from professionals who can provide personalized advice based on individual health conditions.

One potential concern with the ketogenic diet is the possibility of muscle loss. When carbohydrates are restricted, the body may turn to muscle protein as an alternative fuel source, which can lead to muscle wasting if not properly managed. Additionally, some people may experience what is commonly known as "keto flu" during the initial phase of transitioning into ketosis, which can cause symptoms such as fatigue, headache, and nausea. Understanding and managing these potential outcomes is crucial, and healthcare professionals can help individuals navigate through the process.

While a ketogenic diet can be considered safe when followed diligently, it is essential to consult with a healthcare professional to gain a clear understanding of any potential risks, benefits, and individual considerations. They can provide personalized guidance, monitor nutritional status, and ensure the diet is tailored to an individual's specific needs and health conditions.

WHAT ARE THE EFFECTS OF KETO FLU ON YOUR BODY?

When an individual's glucose levels deplete and their body relies on fat for energy, they may experience symptoms known as keto flu. This occurs when the body enters a state called ketosis, where it produces ketones as an alternative fuel source.

During the initial weeks of transitioning to a ketogenic diet, individuals may encounter temporary discomforts commonly referred to as keto flu. These symptoms typically manifest when fasting or maintaining a calorie deficit. Some of the common symptoms include nausea, dizziness, headaches, and difficulties with mental clarity. These symptoms are believed to arise due to the body adjusting to the shift in energy sources and the metabolic changes associated with ketosis.

Although the keto flu can be uncomfortable, it is usually a transient phase that lasts for a short period. The severity and duration of the symptoms can vary among individuals. It's important to note that not everyone experiences the keto flu, and some individuals may transition to ketosis smoothly without any noticeable symptoms.

To alleviate the symptoms and ease the transition into ketosis, there are several strategies that can be employed. Firstly, it's crucial to ensure adequate hydration and electrolyte balance, as the ketogenic diet can increase water and mineral loss. Increasing sodium, potassium, and magnesium intake through food or supplementation can help prevent or alleviate symptoms like dizziness and fatigue.

Additionally, gradually reducing carbohydrate intake instead of making an abrupt change can make the transition smoother and minimize the severity of symptoms. It may also be beneficial to consume small, frequent meals during the initial adaptation period to stabilize blood sugar levels and provide a more gradual adjustment to the new energy source.

Engaging in regular physical exercise, while being mindful of individual energy levels, can also aid in the transition. Exercise can help deplete glycogen stores and facilitate the body's switch to utilizing fat for fuel. However, it's important to listen to your body and make adjustments as needed, as energy levels may fluctuate during the adaptation phase.

Adequate rest and quality sleep are also crucial during this period. The body is undergoing metabolic changes, and sufficient rest can support overall well-being and assist in the adjustment process.

Despite the challenges of the initial adaptation, many individuals find that the benefits of a ketogenic diet outweigh the temporary discomforts. The diet offers a wide range of food options that can be incorporated into a well-rounded meal plan. Some popular choices include keto-friendly cooking oils high in healthy fats, lean meats as a source of protein, low-carbohydrate vegetables, and alternative baking flours that are low in carbs. This assortment of food options makes it easier to select meals that provide sustained nourishment throughout the day while adhering to the principles of the ketogenic diet.

VEGETABLES

Consuming vegetables has indeed been scientifically proven to offer a wide array of health advantages. They are packed with essential nutrients, including vitamins, minerals, and dietary fiber, which are vital for maintaining optimal health and well-being.

One significant benefit of vegetables is their ability to support the body's healing process. The nutrients present in vegetables play a crucial role in supporting immune function and reducing inflammation, which are key factors in the healing process. They provide the body with the necessary vitamins and minerals to repair damaged tissues and fight off infections.

Furthermore, vegetables can help reduce the risk of metabolic disorders. Metabolic disorders such as obesity, type 2 diabetes, and cardiovascular diseases are major health concerns worldwide. Including vegetables in your diet can contribute to weight management and reduce the risk of developing these conditions. Vegetables are generally low in calories and high in fiber, which promotes satiety, aids in weight loss, and helps regulate blood sugar levels.

In addition to their nutritional content, vegetables also play a vital role in promoting gut health. Research has shown that vegetables support the growth and diversity of beneficial gut bacteria. These bacteria, known as probiotics, contribute to digestion, nutrient absorption, and overall gut health. A healthy gut microbiota is associated with numerous health benefits, including improved immune function, reduced risk of inflammatory diseases, and enhanced mental well-being.

Even if you have a dislike for vegetables, it is still beneficial to incorporate them into your diet. There are various ways to make vegetables more appealing and flavorful. For instance, sautéing a variety of vegetables with herbs and spices can enhance their taste and make them more enjoyable to consume. Including raw vegetables like green peppers, carrots, or cucumbers in salads, sandwiches, or stir-fries can add crunch and freshness to your meals.

In situations where obtaining fresh vegetables is challenging, there are alternative options available. Super green powders, made from dehydrated and powdered vegetables, are a convenient way to increase your intake of vegetable antioxidants. They can be easily mixed into smoothies or protein shakes, providing a concentrated dose of nutrients. Additionally, super greens pills or capsules are available as a vegetarian substitute when fresh vegetables are not readily available.

Food	Carb (G)	Serving Size
Cauliflowers	5	1 cup
Onions	9	1 tbsp
Green Beans	10	1 cup
Turnips	6	1 medium
Poblano Peppers	9	1 pepper
Jalapeno Peppers	1	1 pepper
Radishes	3.9	1 cup
Olives	8.5	1 cup
Asparagus	5.3	1 cup

Garlic	1	1 clove
Eggplant	49	1 medium
Celery	3	1 cup
Brussel Sprouts	8	1 cup
Bell peppers	4	1 pepper
Broccoli	6	1 cup
Rhubarb	6	1 cup
Yellow Squash	15	1 medium
Pumpkins	8	1 cup
Mushrooms	8.3	1 cup
Leeks	8	1 cup
Pickles	3.5	1 cup

LEAFY GREENS

Dark leafy greens like spinach and kale are fantastic low-carb options for your diet. They make a great addition to your meals because they are low in carbs and sodium while being rich in essential minerals and vitamins.

These leafy greens provide valuable antioxidants that support your immune system and help reduce metabolic risk factors. However, it's important to note that while incorporating them into your diet is beneficial, no single meal can guarantee the prevention of cancer.

The versatility of leafy greens allows for various preparations to suit your taste and preferences. Here are some ideas:

- Enhance your kale by adding turkey bacon slices for a delicious breakfast.
- Opt for a simple lunch option by enjoying a salad with salmon on top.

- Create the perfect green protein drink by blending greens with your favorite fruits and protein after your workout.
- Make delectable lettuce wraps by chopping chicken and filling lettuce leaves.

Leafy greens offer a wide range of possibilities to include them in your diet. Additionally, most varieties are available throughout the year, making it convenient to stock up on them without straining your budget.

Food	Carbs (G)	Serving Size
Bok Choy	3	1 cup
Butter Lettuce (Bib)	1.2	1 cup
Fennel	6.4	1 cup sliced
Iceberg Lettuce	1.7	1 cup
Rapini (Broccoli Raab)	1	1 cup chopped
Arugula	0.7	1 cup
Swiss chard	13	1 cup chopped
Chicory Greens	1.4	1 cup sliced
Mustard Greens	2.6	1 cup
Endive	1.8	1 cup chopped
Kale	7.3	1 cup

Beet Greens (Beet Root)	7.9	1 cup
Watercress	0.4	1 cup chopped
Romaine lettuce	1.5	1 cup chopped
Turnip Greens	3.9	1 cup chopped
Collard Greens	11	1 cup chopped
Capers	6.7	1 cup
Spinach	8	1 cup

FATS

According to the American Heart Association, the significance of fats in our diet has increased in recent years. They play a vital role in the functioning of our bodies as they contribute to the production of essential fatty acids and fat-soluble vitamins A, D, and E that are necessary for our well-being. Additionally, fats provide energy to our cells and help maintain the warmth of our internal organs.

When following a ketogenic diet, fats should constitute approximately 55 to 60% of your food intake, serving as the primary source of energy. It is advisable to choose fats that provide sustained energy throughout the day.

Incorporating avocados and nuts into your diet is a delicious and convenient way to consume healthy fats. For those with a busy lifestyle, carrying a container of almond butter or peanut butter is a convenient option. To meet your nutritional needs, consider adding MCT oil to your post-workout protein shake.

When it comes to high-temperature cooking, it is recommended to use healthier oils such as extra virgin olive oil, hazelnut oil, or avocado oil. Coconut oil, for instance, not only enhances the flavor of your meals but also provides the necessary fats required for each serving.

Food	Carbs (G)	Serving Size
Butter	0	1 tbsp
MCT Oil	0	1 tbsp
Almond Oil	0	1 tbsp
Soybean Oil	0	1 tbsp
Ghee butter	0	1 tbsp
Coconut Oil	0	1 tbsp
Extra Virgin Olive Oil	0	1 tbsp
Avocado Oil	0	1 tbsp
Flaxseed Oil	0	1 tbsp

FRUITS

If you're following the keto diet, incorporating fruit into your meals can be a wonderful alternative to sugar and sweeteners. By reducing your reliance on sugary treats, you can maintain balanced blood sugar levels.

Fortunately, there is an abundance of fruit options to choose from. Bananas and mangoes, in particular, are rich in vitamins and minerals, making them suitable for consumption during any mealtime. Bananas are packed with potassium, an electrolyte essential for regulating blood pressure, and vitamin B6, which our bodies are unable to produce. Various studies have shown that vitamin B6 can enhance cognitive function and alleviate nausea and vomiting in expectant mothers.

Mangoes, on the other hand, are a high-fiber fruit brimming with antioxidants. They aid in preventing rapid sugar absorption into the bloodstream and assist in regulating insulin levels. Remarkably, a single cup of mango provides ten times the recommended daily intake of vitamin C.

Even while in ketosis, you can still enjoy a touch of sweetness by incorporating your preferred fruits into your diet.

Food	Carbs (G)	Serving Size
Watermelon	11	1 cup
Avocados	17	1
Bananas	27	1 medium
Pears	35	1 large
Apple	25	1 medium
Blackberries	14	1 cup
Coconut (Flesh)	12.9	1 cup
Cranberries	13.2	1 cup
Cantaloupe	45	1 cup cubed
Kiwi	10	1 fruit
Lemons	19.8	1 cup sliced
Limes	7.6	1 cup sliced
Mango	24.7	1 cup sliced
Raspberries	14.7	1 cup
Peach	17	1 large
Strawberries	12.7	1 cup sliced
Pineapple	19.5	1 cup sliced

Plums	7.54	1 fruit
Grapes	16	1 cup
Blueberries	21.4	1 cup
Tomatoes	4.8	1 medium
Orange	22	1 large

MEATS AND POULTRY

Protein plays a vital role as the fundamental building block of the body. It contributes to the maintenance of bone density and strength, as well as the repair of internal organs and tissues. Alongside its high protein content, lean meats and poultry offer a plethora of other health advantages.

When adhering to the keto diet, it is recommended that protein should account for 30-35 percent of your daily caloric intake. Consuming moderate amounts of chicken or steak, for instance, can promote a sense of fullness and satiate your hunger.

Creatine, a naturally occurring substance produced by the body, can also be found in red foods such as steak. This amino acid aids in increasing muscle mass and providing energy to the body. Including lean steak in your diet can effectively contribute to muscle development.

Food	Carbs (G)	Serving Size
Bacon (Cooked)	0.2	1 slice
Italian Sausage	3	1 link
Ground Beef	0	4 oz
Hot Dog	2	1 link
Duck Liver	1.6	1 liver (44g)
Lamb	0	4 oz
Lamb Chops	0	6 oz
Breakfast Sausage	0	1 link
Bratwurst	2	1 link
Pork	0	6 oz
Top Sirloin	0	4 oz
Ground Turkey, Chicken	0	4 oz
Deli meats: chicken, turkey, ham, pastrami, etc.	0.7	1 oz
Veal	0	4 oz
Bison	0	4 oz

SEAFOOD

Seafood serves as a popular protein option, with salmon standing out due to its abundance of essential vitamins and minerals. It is particularly beneficial for vegetarians and individuals who avoid red meat and poultry, as it contains valuable nutrients like omega-3 fatty acids, iron, and vitamins B and D.

Research suggests that fish is a favorable choice for weight loss, as it is low in fat and calories while providing ample protein. Additionally, incorporating fish into one's diet can support brain function, promote heart health, and reduce the risk of stroke.

The versatility of fish, such as salmon, is notable as it can be prepared quickly, taking less than 20 minutes. Pairing it with a refreshing salad of leafy greens, steamed vegetables, or even guacamole makes for a delightful supper option.

Food	Carb (B)	Serving Size
Salmon	0	3 oz
Sardines	0	1 small
Squid	2.6	3 oz
Trout	0	3 oz
Tuna (Bluefin)	0	3 oz
Octopus	3.7	3 oz
Oysters (Pacific)	2.5	1 medium
Clams	4.4	3 oz
Flounder	0	3 oz
Herring	0	3 oz
Mackerel	0	3 oz
Scallops	4.6	3 oz
Shrimp	1	3 oz
Mussels	6	3 oz

NUTS AND SEEDS

Nuts and seeds have gained significant popularity as snacks among those following the keto diet. They offer a range of health benefits, thanks to their omega-3 fatty acid content, which can be found in nuts, avocados, and fish.

Incorporating nuts and seeds into a low-carbohydrate diet is important. For example, walnuts contain approximately 16.5 grams of fat per serving, while pumpkin seeds contain only 5 grams. Enjoying moderate portions of nuts and seeds throughout the day can provide a convenient energy boost, but it's important not to overindulge. While nuts and seeds are rich in omega-3 fats, they also contain carbohydrates.

To make the most of nuts and seeds, it's recommended to prepare them in small portions before each meal. This ensures that you can fully benefit from their nutritional value.

Food	Carbs (G)	Serving Size
Sunflower Seeds	28	1 cup
Walnuts (Chopped)	16	1 cup
Peanut Butter	8	1 tbsp
Peanuts	24	1 cup
Chia Seeds	48	1 cup
Flax Seeds	49	1 cup
Hazelnuts	23	1 cup
Pistachios	34	1 cup
Poppy Seeds	39	1 cup
Pumpkin Seeds	34	1 cup
Pecans	15	1 cup
Pine Nuts	18	1 cup
Almond Butter	9	1 tbsp
Almonds	30	1 cup
Brazil Nuts	15	1 cup
Cashews	39	1 cup
Hemp Seeds	48	1 cup
Macadamia Nuts	19	1 cup

PLANT-BASED PROTEINS

If you choose to abstain from consuming meat, you have the option to substitute it with plant-based alternatives. Alongside vegan protein powders, you can incorporate plant-based sources of protein, such as tempeh, edamame, tofu, and beans, into your main meals.

Tempeh is created through the fermentation of soybeans and provides 8 grams of carbohydrates and 33 grams of protein per cup. Tofu, derived from curdled milk, contains four grams of carbs along with its notable protein and carbohydrate content.

The keto diet doesn't have to pose challenges for vegans. During peak seasons, most supermarkets offer vegan burgers crafted from beans or soy.

Food	Carbs (G)	Serving Size
Lentils	40	1 cup
Chickpeas	45	1 cup
Tempeh	13	1 cup
Tofu	4	1 cup
Quinoa	28	1 cup

Seitan (Wheat Gluten)	13.6	1 cup
Spirulina	27	1 cup

DAIRY AND EGGS

Eggs and dairy products are excellent choices for a ketogenic diet due to their rich nutrient profile. These dairy products are widely available in most grocery stores and offer delightful flavors. Dairy products provide a good number of proteins and fats, making them versatile for incorporating multiple macronutrients into your diet when tracking calories.

One notable option is goat cheese, which contains zero carbs and six grams of fat per ounce. Blue cheese, on the other hand, has five grams of fat and seven grams of carbohydrates per ounce.

For those who are lactose intolerant or follow a vegan diet, there are alternative options such as oats, almonds, hemp, or soy. However, it's important to note that some of these alternatives may have higher sugar and protein content compared to cow's milk, as indicated by studies.

Eggs are low in carbohydrates (6%), but they are rich in protein (6g) and fat (2g). To save time when preparing family dinners, it's convenient to pre-prepare larger quantities of these ingredients.

If you prefer plant-based alternatives or avoid eggs altogether, there are simple substitutes available. Silken tofu can be used as an egg replacement in baking, while regular tofu can be used in other instances.

Food	Carbs (G)	Serving Size
Eggs (Grade A, Large, White)	6	1 large egg
Almond Milk	3.4	1 cup
Sour Cream	1	1 tbsp
Goat Cheese	0	1 oz
Soy Milk	8	1 cup
Oat Milk	16	1 cup
Rice Milk	22	1 cup
Cream Cheese	0.8	1 tbsp
Half-and-Half	0.7	1 tbsp
Blue Cheese	0.7	1 oz
Parmesan Cheese (Hard)	1	1 oz
Heavy Cream (Whipped)	6.5	1 cup

BEVERAGES

Both your beverage and food choices play a significant role in the keto diet. It is essential to stay properly hydrated during the initial stages of the ketogenic diet to avoid experiencing symptoms of keto flu. According to the recommendations from the National Academies of Sciences, Engineering, and Medicine, men should aim to drink 131 ounces of water per day, while women should aim for 95 ounces per day to support their keto diets. Adequate hydration will help replenish and nourish your body.

In the context of the keto diet, there are a few exceptions when it comes to beverage options. While attempting to lose weight, it is advisable to avoid soda as it is not conducive to your dietary goals.

When it comes to alcohol consumption while on the ketogenic diet, moderation is key. You don't have to give up your social life in order to prioritize your health.

Traditional beer is generally not recommended for individuals following the keto diet due to its high sugar and carbohydrate content, which can hinder weight loss efforts. However, certain variations of the keto diet may allow for the consumption of light beer in moderation.

During social gatherings, it is advisable to opt for clear spirits like vodka or gin. Rum, for instance, tends to have a higher sugar content compared to vodka. These spirits can be enjoyed straight, on the rocks, or in a cocktail, depending on your preference.

Food	Carbs (G)	Serving Size
Light Beer (Michelob Ultra)	2.6	12 fl. oz
Black Tea (Brewed/Unsweetened)	0	8 fl. oz
Crystal Light	0	8 fl. oz
White Tea (Brewed/Unsweetened)	0	8 fl. oz
Green Tea (Brewed/Unsweetened)	0	8 fl. oz
Cranberry Juice (Tropicana)	35	8 fl. oz

Gatorade	35	32 fl. oz
Coffee	0	8 fl. oz
Soda Water, Seltzer, Mineral Water	0	8 fl. oz
Unsweetened Iced Tea (Lipton)	0	8 fl. oz
White Wine	4	5 fl. oz
Orange Juice (Minute Maid)	27	32 fl. oz
Bone Broth	0.6	8 fl. oz
Diet Soda (Coke Zero)	5	12 fl. oz
Gin	0	1.5 fl. oz
Powerade	22	32 fl. oz
Water	0	8 fl. oz
Red Wine	4	5 fl. oz
Pineapple Juice (Dole)	32	8 fl. oz
Tequila (80 proof)	0	1.5 fl. oz
Vodka	0	1.5 fl. oz

FLOURS FOR BAKING

You can indulge in delicious baked goods regardless of your dietary restrictions. By substituting all-purpose, maize, and wheat flour with keto-friendly alternatives, you can still relish comfort food using coconut, almond, sunflower seed, or flax meal flours.

Instead of relying on traditional high-carbohydrate options, consider incorporating protein balls into your routine. These nutrient-packed treats are rich in protein and can provide the energy you need for workouts or serve as a wholesome snack. Adopting a new eating regimen doesn't mean sacrificing enjoyment; it simply means making smarter choices.

Food	Carbs (G)	Serving Size
Oat Flour	68	1 cup
Cocoa Powder	50	1 cup
Chia Seed Flour	24	1 cup
Soy Flour	43	1 cup
Macadamia Flour	36	1 cup
Almond Flour	24	1 cup

Coconut Flour	65	1 cup
Hazelnut Flour	23	1 cup
Almond Meal	24	1 cup
Ground Flaxseed	49	1 cup

SWEETENERS

Numerous sweeteners are not permitted on the keto diet, which can be disappointing for individuals who enjoy adding sugar to their coffee and tea. While sugar might be restricted, there are still alternatives available to add sweetness to your preferred foods and beverages.

By incorporating sweeteners such as stevia or xylitol in moderation, you can effectively manage your craving for sweetness. Stevia has gained popularity as a widely used sugar substitute in both restaurants and households. Xylitol, often found in sugar-free gums, is another substitute that doesn't impact blood sugar levels differently than stevia.

Another natural sweetener and Southeast Asian superfood known as lou han gou, or monk fruit, can be a great choice. It has been recognized as a safe sugar substitute by the FDA, falling under the category of Generally Recognized as Safe (GRAS).

Food	Carbs (G)	Serving Size
Erythritol	4	1 tsp
Sweet'n Low	1	per pack
Stevia	0	per packet
Splenda	0	per packet
Monk Fruit Sweetener (In the Raw)	1	per packet
Sucralose	0	1 tsp
Equal	0	per packet

HERBS AND SPICES

Improving your diet doesn't have to be a daunting task. One simple way to enhance your meals is by incorporating keto-friendly herbs and spices. These flavorful additions are typically low in carbs and can bring new life to otherwise plain dishes, such as ground turkey or grilled meats. To ensure you're maintaining a low carbohydrate intake, it's important to carefully review food labels.

Consider trying Chinese Five Spice, which offers a delightful blend of sweetness and spiciness, making it an excellent complement to savory chicken dishes. Another versatile option is Adobo, a popular seasoning found in Portuguese, Puerto Rican, Mexican, and Filipino cuisines. Adobo spices infuse meats like steak, chicken, pork, and fish with a distinctive and delicious flavor.

Furthermore, you may already have keto-friendly herbs and spices in your kitchen, such as cinnamon, mint, cayenne pepper, and ginger. These ingredients can be easily incorporated into your cooking, adding depth and zest to your meals while remaining consistent with a keto-friendly approach.

Food	Carb (G)	Serving Size
Cinnamon	5	1 tbsp
Chili Powder	4	1 tbsp
Cilantro	0	1 tbsp
Rosemary	2	1 tbsp
Basil	1	2 tbsp
Tarrago	2.4	1 tbsp
Chinese 5 Spice	4.2	1 4.2
Mint	5	2 tbsp
Adobo (Goya)	0	1 tbsp
Garam Masala	7	1 tbsp
Parsley	0.2	1 tbsp
Cayenne	3	1 tbsp
Thyme	9.6	1 tbsp
Paprika	3.7	1 tbsp
Garlic Powder (Lawry's)	1	1 tbsp

CONDIMENTS

While following the keto diet, it is important to be mindful of condiments and their ingredients. Although the use of condiments is not entirely restricted, it requires careful label reading to identify hidden sugars and chemicals. For instance, Hunt's ketchup often contains high-fructose corn syrup. To adhere to the keto diet, it is advisable to search for low-sugar alternatives or create your own sugar-free version using low-carb ingredients.

Condiments like salad dressings and ketchup are commonly employed to enhance the taste of meals. However, it is essential to consider the cumulative impact of these additions, especially when frequently using ranch dressing on salads and chicken dishes. To enhance the nutritional value of your salad, opting for a vinaigrette dressing is a better choice. Additionally, keto-friendly condiments such as mayonnaise, Sriracha, or mustard can be used to add flavor to your meals without significantly affecting your carbohydrate macros.

Food	Carbs (G)	Serving Size
Sriracha (Huy Fong Foods)	3	1 tbsp
Sugar-free Steak Sauce (G Hughes)	1	1 tbsp
Vinaigrette	0.4	1 tbsp
Mayonnaise	0	1 tbsp
Sugar-free BBQ Sauce (G Hughes)	1	1 tbsp
Liquid Aminos (Soy Sauce Alternative)	0.1	1 tbsp
Mustard	1	1 tbsp
Marinara Sauce	10	.5 cup
Hot Sauce (Frank's RedHot Original)	0	1 tbsp
Kimchi	3.6	1 cup
Unsweetened Ketchup (Primal Kitchen)	2	1 tbsp

CONCLUSION

The keto diet offers numerous benefits, including weight loss and an increase in good cholesterol levels. However, it is important to seek guidance from a trained dietitian, nutritionist, or consult with your doctor before starting any dietary regimen.

Irrespective of whether you decide to modify your eating habits, there are plenty of low-carb food choices accessible. Achieving your weight-loss goals requires discipline, but maintaining good health should always be a priority.

Printed in Great Britain
by Amazon